W9-BBJ-667

Faces of Osteoporosis

AMELIA DAVIS

Demos

Demos Medical Publishing, LLC, 386 Park Avenue South, New York,
New York 10016

Visit out website at www.demosmedpub.com

Book designed by Milieu Design Studio, www.milieudesignstudio.com

Art direction by Rebecca Martinez, www.rebeccamartinez.com

Library of Congress Cataloging-in-Publication Data

Davis, Amelia.
  Faces of osteoporosis / Amelia Davis.
    p. cm.
  ISBN-10: 1-932603-62-X
  ISBN-13: 978-1932-60362-0
  1. Osteoporosis--Popular works. 2. Osteoporosis--Patients--Biography. I.
Title.
  RC931.O73.D38 2006
  616.7´16--dc22
                                                      2005028901

For my two nieces

MADELEINE AND ABIGAIL AND THE CHILDREN OF THE FUTURE

Contents

Introduction

UNITED STATES SENATOR
DIANNE FEINSTEIN

Dear Friends,

When many of us hear the word osteoporosis, a picture of an old, frail, hunched woman comes to mind. This is an all too common image. However, osteoporosis affects men and women, young and old, from all ethnic groups and walks of life. If we are to begin to reduce the numbers of people who have fractures resulting from low bone mass or osteoporosis, we need to see ourselves and our loved ones in the many faces of osteoporosis.

Millions of Americans have low bone mass or osteoporosis. It is very likely that all of us will be touched by this preventable disease – it may be our mother or father, grandmother or grandfather, friend or other family member. As I can tell you from personal experience, the impact of a fracture can change the course of your life immeasurably.

Our first challenge is to recognize that no one is exempt from taking steps to improve his or her bone health. This important book documents the stories of people who are living with osteoporosis. The book will help you understand the silent and devastating impact of the disease. I hope that you will learn from these brave individuals who share their stories with you. We must educate and empower people through knowledge. Together, I hope we can eliminate osteoporosis as a major health problem.

Foreword

CALIFORNIA STATE SENATOR
ELAINE ALQUIST

As the founder of the California Osteoporoses Prevention and Education (COPE) program which began in 1999, it is with great pleasure that I introduce *Faces of Osteoporosis* to you. The profiles of osteoporosis that you will see in the following pages are a compelling reminder that osteoporosis can affect anyone.

After reading this book, you will no longer see osteoporosis only in the face of a stooped, older woman, who walks with a cane. Rather, you will learn about:

Perry Ann who is only forty. She's climbed some of the highest peaks in North America and northern Europe, plays tennis, eats a healthy diet, never smoked, never broken a bone but has low bone mass, a possible precursor to osteoporosis. Could be genetics...could be a childhood diet lacking in adequate calcium and vitamin D.

Renea who volunteered to be a test patient for a class of technicians learning how to use bone density screening equipment. Imagine her surprise when she was told that she had severe osteoporosis! Renea had recently broken bones, but that was because of a car accident... or did her bones break because they couldn't withstand the impact from the accident because they were brittle with osteoporosis? For the last 30 years, Renea was taking medication to control epilepsy; she was also post-menopausal. She did not know that treatment for one disease could put her at risk for osteoporosis.

Andrew who was only 9 when he fell from a swing and was taken to the hospital. It turned out he had three compression fractures in his back, and his bones showed that he had osteoporosis.

As a middle-aged woman, I know and live with the risks of osteoporosis every day. There are many faces of osteoporosis. Don't wait until you see it. Eat a balanced diet with adequate calcium and vitamin D. Exercise. And remember, osteoporosis is detectable, highly preventable, and treatable.

Acknowledgments

I would like to thank all the people featured in this book.

Lynn Trowbridge rallied for me and this book. I thank her for getting the ball rolling and helping make this book a reality.

Faces of Osteoporosis would not have been possible without a grant from The State of California and UCSF.

Special thanks go to Pam Ford from COPE and UCSF and to Kathleen Cody and Beverley Tracewell from FORE.

I am grateful to Elizabeth Davis, my sister, and Luis Penalver, my brother-in-law, for their support and professional advice.

Jim Marshall once again offered unquestioning help and support.

Kirk Anspach did all the printing of my photographs and offered encouragement for my work.

I could not do what I do without the unwavering support and love of Bonita Passarelli.

Osteoporosis

FOUNDATION OF OSTEOPOROSIS
RESEARCH AND EDUCATION

Osteoporosis is a bone disease with a complicated sound-
ing name. Simply speaking, osteoporosis describes bones
("osteo") that are relatively porous ("porosis") compared
to normal bones. People with osteoporosis have bones
that are weaker than normal because there is low bone
mass and poor structural integrity. Usually poor structural
integrity is associated with low bone mass, but this may not
always be the case. Having weak bones puts people with
osteoporosis at risk for broken bones or fractures
especially at the hip, wrist, and spine, but also in other
parts of their body. Like high blood pressure or high
cholesterol, osteoporosis is a silent disease—that is, until
a fracture happens. Fractures are the most dangerous part
of osteoporosis. Fractures can cause pain, disability, and
loss of independence and lead to premature death. The
most common fractures from osteoporosis are compression fractures of the vertebrae (bones of the spine). These
fractures cause the curved back (kyphosis) seen in people
with advanced osteoporosis. Hip fractures can lead to
isolation, loss of mobility, and even death.

Osteoporosis is not part of the normal aging process. Osteoporosis is a disease that is preventable and treatable. We all face many health risks, and osteoporosis should be at the top of your list to discuss with your doctor.

HERE ARE SOME FACTS ABOUT OSTEOPOROSIS:
• In the United States alone, there are 30 million women and 14 million men with osteoporosis or at risk for osteoporosis. Many of these individuals have not been diagnosed and are not being treated.
• One out of two women and one out of five men over 50 years of age will suffer a fracture because of osteoporosis.
• Osteoporosis leads to 300,000 hip fractures each year; 20%–30% of people with hip fractures will die from related complications within one year; half will permanently lose their independence; 20% will require long-term nursing care.
• Osteoporosis affects more women than breast cancer, uterine cancer, and colon cancer combined.
• Osteoporosis affects people from all ethnic groups.
• There are safe and effective medicines that can help prevent and treat osteoporosis.

BONE
Bone is a living, growing tissue that is constantly renewing itself or being remodeled. Remodeling is an ongoing cycle of old bone being broken down and new, healthy bone being formed. This is a normal and important process that maintains the proper functioning of your body by keeping bones strong and providing adequate calcium and other minerals for all the body's tissues. Between birth and about age 30, your body is building a strong skeleton by creating new bone faster than it is being broken down. During this time, children need enough calcium, weight-bearing exercise, and normal hormone levels to build the strongest possible bones. By age 30, you have developed the strongest bones you are going to have during your lifetime. This point is called your **peak adult bone mass.**

For the next 10–20 years, unless something happens to disturb the remodeling process, your bone density will remain constant. The cycle of bone remodeling is balanced and important in repairing minor damage that occurs to bones in everyday life.

Hormones are important to the bone remodeling process. When women reach menopause and their estrogen levels decline, this affects the rate of bone building. The bone remodeling process becomes unbalanced and women are subject to rapid bone loss. While men typically build more bone than women when they are children, they may also experience bone loss. This may be due to decreasing male hormone (testosterone) levels or for other reasons.

Diagnosis

Osteoporosis occurs when the system of remodeling becomes unbalanced and either too much bone is broken down or not enough bone is replaced. This causes the bone density to decline allowing bones to break more easily. A simple test is available to check for osteoporosis. Dual Energy X-Ray Absorptiometry (DEXA) allows doctors to measure your bone mineral density. The test is simple and painless, and although it uses X-rays, the amount of radiation is very small and does not pose a health hazard. Based on criteria set by the World Health Organization, osteoporosis can be diagnosed when the T-score (a measure of how far the BMD is from normal young people) is 2.5 standard deviations below normal.

One negative standard deviation is equal to a 10–12% reduction in bone mineral density and this increases risk of fracture by two to three times.

Treatment and prevention

Osteoporosis can rob you of your lifestyle and independence. Early detection of osteoporosis and monitoring your bone health are important. If you do not have osteoporosis now, there are many things that you can do to prevent getting it later. If you do have osteoporosis, there are many things you can do to keep your bones from getting weaker or breaking. However, there are simple changes that you can begin making today that can improve your bone health for a lifetime.

A diet rich in calcium along with regular weight-bearing exercise are essential for bone health. Talk with your doctor about your diet and lifestyle and whether additional supplements of calcium and vitamin D are recommended. Your doctor can also advise you on an exercise routine. Most importantly, as the Surgeon General says, you are never too young or too old to improve your bone health. What is most important is beginning the lifetime work of building and keeping strong bones.

Faces of Osteoporosis

Hi, my name is Amy, and I'm eleven years old going into the sixth grade. I love animals! I have a bird named Tweety and a bunny named Daisy. I jazz-dance with groups for competitions. I enjoy listening to all kinds of music. I also love hanging out with my friends. I'm a normal pre-teen girl except for my bones.

The first time I remember I broke a bone was over Christmas break. I was walking our neighbor's dog named Cooper. Cooper saw another dog and ran after it. When I didn't let go he pulled me down, and I broke my wrist and shoulder blade (scapula). It really hurt and I cried a lot. My cast for my wrist was green and blue, and then for my scapula I had to wear a sling.

I broke my wrist again at dance class when I fell off a stool. I didn't cry as much this time. My mom said as soon as she saw how I was holding my arm she knew it was broken. This time I got a blue cast.

A month later I broke my foot when I was running. My shoes were not tied and I fell out of them. All my friends were there—it was kind of embarrassing. It didn't hurt as bad as the wrist did. I got a red cast to match my fifth grade teacher's who broke her ankle a couple weeks before. I had the best doctor! Dr. Sawyer is a pediatric orthopedic doctor. I have had many tests. Dr. Sawyer and her office manager Rita took very good care of me. That's all the bones I remember breaking.

My parents told me of the other times when I broke my bones. I was too young to remember. I was born with two broken legs but didn't know at first. My mom said I cried a lot when she would change my diaper. Mom was told that it was probably a dislocated hip and it would heal fast. At six weeks old I had a body cast on. This is when my parents found out that I had two broken legs at birth. Since one leg didn't heal correctly it broke again easily.

When I was three years old I was running around the house with my older brother, Mathew. I fell and my brother couldn't stop and stepped on me. My parents found out a day later that my collarbone (clavicle) was broken. This is a bone that cannot be put in a cast so I had a sling. That is all the bones I have broken and I hope I don't break any more!

Our family just recently found out I have osteogenesis imperfecta (brittle bone disease). This means I cannot play any contact sports and I need to be careful when I dance.

I don't feel any different but maybe a little special.

What drew me to Amy immediately was her openness and acceptance of osteoporosis at such a young age.

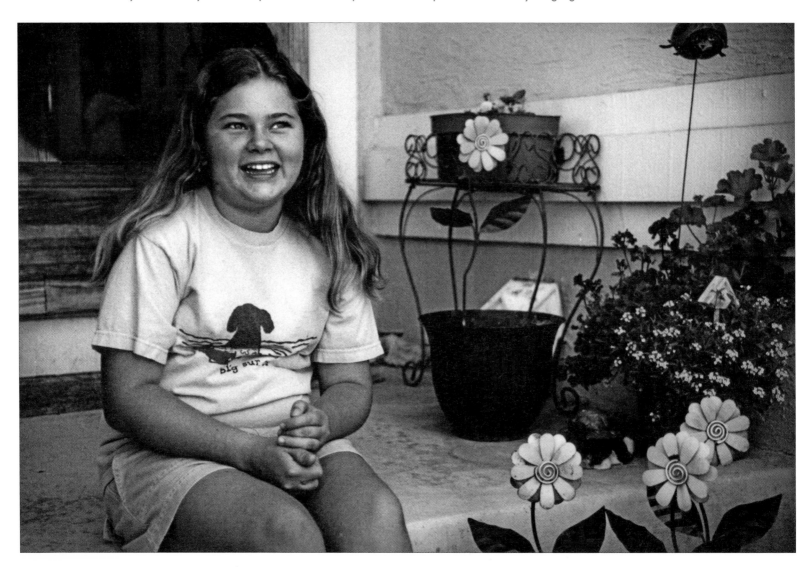

Amy is lucky to have a mother that is so supportive.

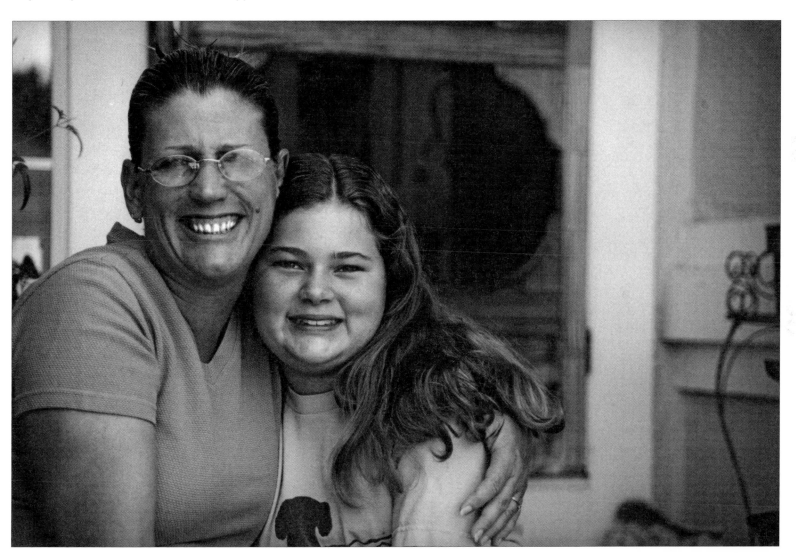

These two lovely seniors were both born in the north- ern provinces of Russia. They appear to be the picture of health, and both belie their four-score-plus and four-score-and-ten-plus years. Boris does have the more traditional, slightly kyphotic appearance to his profile but this is not really remarkable given his age. Imagine our surprise when we recently conducted bone density tests on them and discovered what incredibly low bone density they had.

Certainly my curiosity was aroused, and this prompted me to interview Marina. This very bright and articulate woman surprised me yet further. My first question was "What was your childhood like?" Her response did not clear up my confusion. She said "I was raised on a farm, drank a lot of milk every day, and worked physi- cally very hard."

We continued our conversation while I tossed around this information looking for the answer to the puzzle. Then it struck me: vitamin D.

While clearly they were getting adequate calcium and exer- cise during the bone-building years (9–20 approximately),

it was certainly reasonable to suspect that although they had the basic ingredients for good strong bones, they were probably missing the catalyst to convert the calcium to bone.

Science tells us that the more northerly the latitude the less effective the sun's rays are in inducing the skin to produce vitamin D. Compounding this problem, the northern provinces of Russia experience very little if any sun for long stretches of the winter months. In addition to all of this, the style of the day, for Russian women in particular, was to be all bundled up with very little skin actually exposed to the sun when it did penetrate the Rus- sian darkness.

And so, despite what appeared to be a healthy childhood in many ways, these two senior Russians are experiencing osteoporosis, probably induced by a lack of vitamin D dur- ing those crucial bone-building years of their childhood. A very different osteoporosis story.

I met Boris briefly at the Russian Senior Center and felt as if I had known him for a long time. It shocked me to learn his true age.

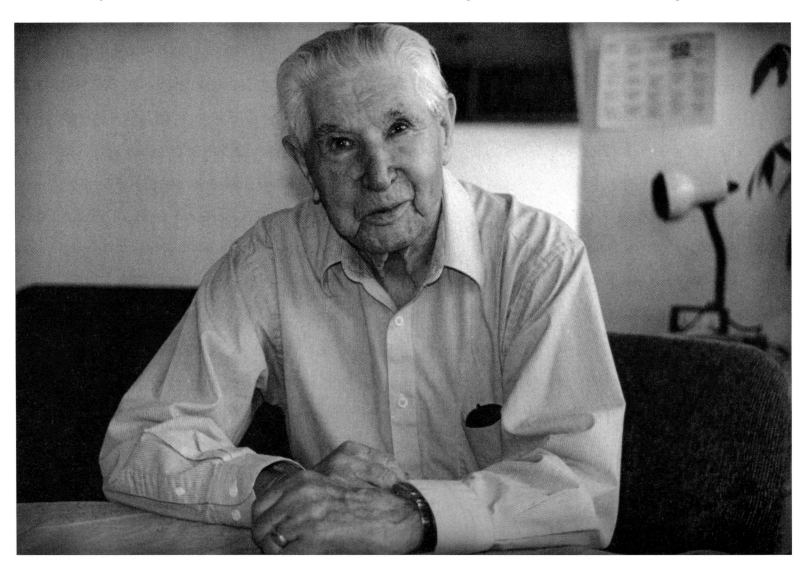

Such an elegant, educated and open woman.

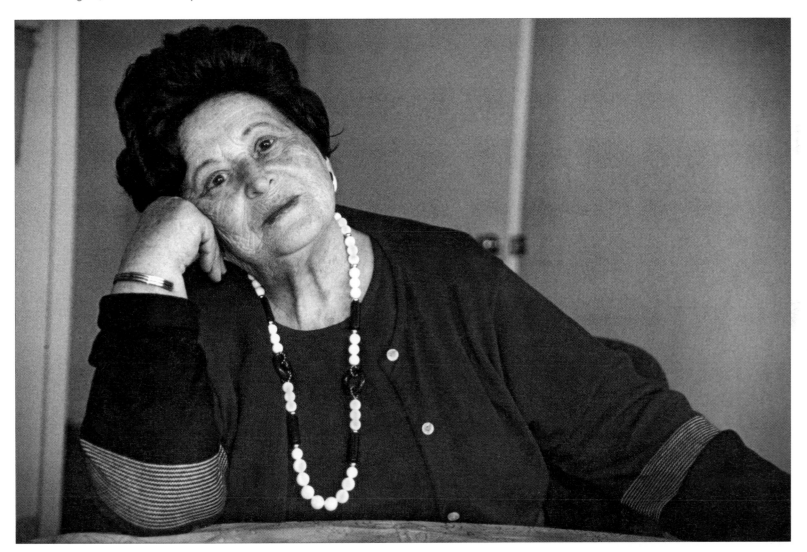

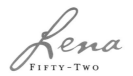

Lena
FIFTY-TWO

My Mom and I are a lot alike. People say that of my three siblings and me, I am the one who takes after Mom in looks and character. It's a good thing; Mom was always full of energy, a caring person, compassionate and generous when she was in her prime. She was humble when people complimented her on how she never looked her age.

Mom was strong. She and Dad ran a small mom-and-pop grocery store together from 1948 until all of us kids were done with college and settled in our own lives. Mom would get up at 3:00 a.m. to get things ready at the store, putting out the produce, filling the shelves. She would come back home at 7:30 a.m. to wake us kids up to get ready for school. The rest of the day would be filled with cooking our lunch and dinner and running us to school and back. In between she would be the checker at the register for the shoppers. She also baby-sat the three kids next door while the parents went to work. We six kids spent a lot of time together, playing while Mom and Dad kept an eye on us and on the store. They retired in 1976 only because the neighborhood where the store was situated had deteriorated and it was no longer a safe environment.

She is still strong. But now she is strong in spirit and weak physically. When I began my job as a pharmaceutical representative for Wyeth Laboratories, Mom was disappointed that I would not be sitting at a desk in an office;

she just could not catch me during the day any time she wanted. It was the age before cell phones! It was a good job for me and I did well. I did it for twenty years and learned all about women's health, including osteoporosis, menopause, and their consequences. I detailed doctors and nurses about prevention and treatment of osteoporosis. I tried to pass this information on to Mom, but she was the victim of media scare tactics just like millions of other women are in English and in the Chinese language. No way was she going to take anything that would give her breast cancer! She would rather die of a heart attack, she'd say. When I warned her about kyphosis she sarcastically said old people are supposed to look like that. She was, and still is very stubborn; listening to reason is not in her cards.

Dad passed away of congestive heart failure. Mom took care of him day and night for a whole year as he deteriorated right before our eyes. He was strong, too. Even though he was physically exhausted and suffered myriad problems, his attitude was to live life to the fullest until the very end. When he passed away, Mom literally looked twenty years older. That year had exhausted her as well.

I knew that osteoporosis ran in her family. We are Asian and are at high risk anyway, but I could tell that Mom had lost quite a few inches in height. She was always taller

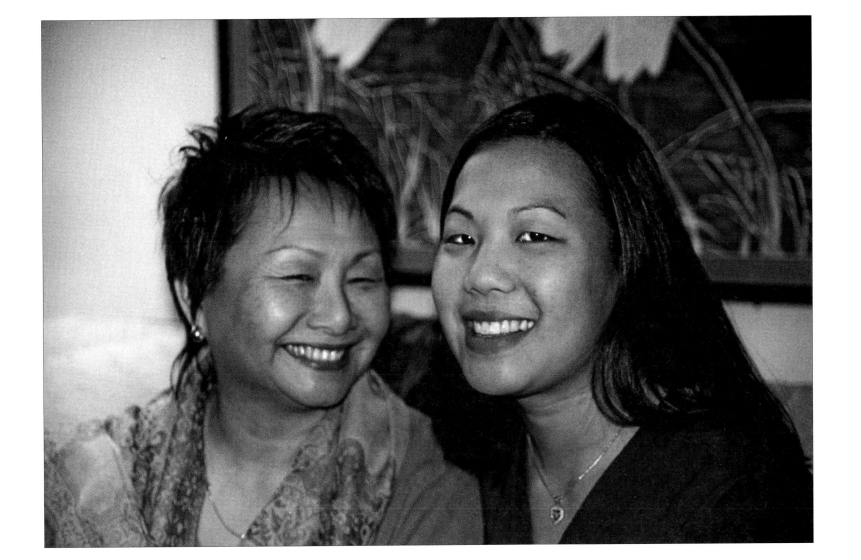

than I, at five feet one or so. I'm only five feet tall, but Mom is now about four feet nine. She suffered a fall two years ago. She did not break any bones but she complained that her back hurt terribly. The doctor said there was nothing to do but rest and take pain medication. Within six months my mother, who had been strong and straight, was now bent over like a weeping willow and could barely walk without the aid of a walker or cane or holding on to another person.

This 83-year-old woman who had the strength of a warrior has now a changed disposition. She, the indefatigable socialite, now refuses to attend most social events because "she does not look good, her clothes do not fit right." She is cranky, demanding, and miserably lonely, even though she has a caretaker twenty-four hours a day, neighbors who visit, and kids who take turns to care for her each weekend when the caretaker has a day off. She is terribly unhappy with the way she feels, the way she looks, and her limited lifestyle. We are looking into treatment to stop the bone loss, but she changes her mind daily about whether or not to do so. There is nothing we can do to reverse the kyphosis. She has just about given up for herself, but she did say to me that since I am far more educated, younger, and know better, that I should take my own advice and prevent the same things from happening to me. You bet I will.

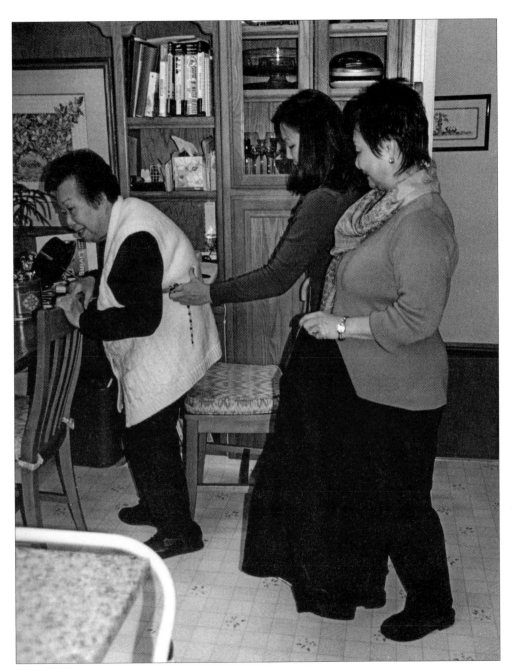

Three generations: Lena, her mom, and her daughter.

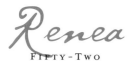

Renea
FIFTY-TWO

Osteoporosis a disease of the bone that I, along with many others, associated with the elderly. Especially those who had visual signs of the disease—a hump in their back, walking severely bent over with a cane, or unable to stand up straight.

My attitude and perception changed when I learned that I had osteoporosis! I was hit by a car in February 2003, resulting in the need to stay off of my feet for several months while the broken bones healed. It was after this accident that I participated in a class that taught technicians how to use the bone-density testing machines and prepare and read test results. As a result of participating in this activity, I learned that I had a severe case of osteoporosis. It was then that I knew I had to do something to strengthen my bones to avoid the other debilitating characteristics that come with the disease. At the same time, I began a search for the reasons I developed osteoporosis. After all, I didn't have a small frame and I wasn't in one of the higher-risk ethnic groups.

In January 2003, I was asked to volunteer as a member of the Finance Committee for the Foundation for Osteoporosis Research and Education (FORE). As a committee member, I learned of the campaign to inform men and women in their thirties of the disease and its impact. The underlying message throughout this campaign was that osteoporosis is not something that we should expect or accept as part of the normal aging process. Instead, with proper diet, exercise, and the right information,

osteoporosis is a disease whose affects can be minimized or completely deterred.

I have never been one to take calcium supplements, nor drink milk, other than with cereal. I exercised daily and ate healthy foods. However, I was post-menopausal and had been taking medication to control epilepsy for thirty years. I enjoyed an ample daily dose of caffeinated beverages. In combination, prolonged use of anti-seizure medication, minimal intake of calcium and vitamin D, and my daily intake of caffeine contributed to the decrease in bone mass.

Today, I purposely find ways to ingest calcium in the form of calcium with vitamin D supplements, yogurt, and cheese. In addition, I look for calcium in its natural fruit and vegetable sources—like calcium-enriched orange juice, almonds, sunflower seeds, and leafy green vegetables. Although I cannot participate in aerobics, I can walk and use exercise equipment that helps to build muscle and bone mass.

I no longer think of osteoporosis as an older persons' disease. I take every opportunity to share with the twenty- and thirty-somethings that they are at risk if they don't eat right and keep themselves in shape. I've always been a catalyst for change. It's great to know that, unlike many of the other diseases we hear about today, there is something that we can do to alter the results. Keep moving!

I learned an important message from Renea: be aware of other medications you are on, because over time, they could contribute to you getting osteoporosis.

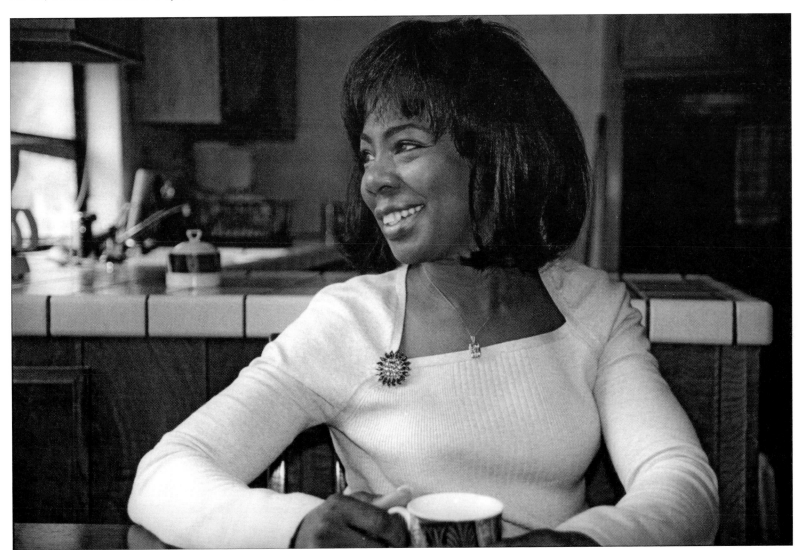

It took me by surprise when Eric shared with me that he has osteoporosis, because he is a successful yoga instructor.

Eric

FORTY-FIVE

When Amelia asked if I'd be a part of this project, I felt
odd. This was in part due to being a bit shy about photographs of myself. But what was behind those odd feelings
was realizing I hadn't thought much about my condition.
In the few years since testing revealed low bone density,
diet and lifestyle changes have been my efforts. And I don't
have my mother around anymore to be a visual reminder
of osteoporosis. So this was a reminder to be grateful for
the health I've been experiencing the last couple of years.
I'm also reminded of how strong-spirited my mother was,
and many of us living with these conditions share that joy
of living.

Howard found out this very day that he has osteoporosis.

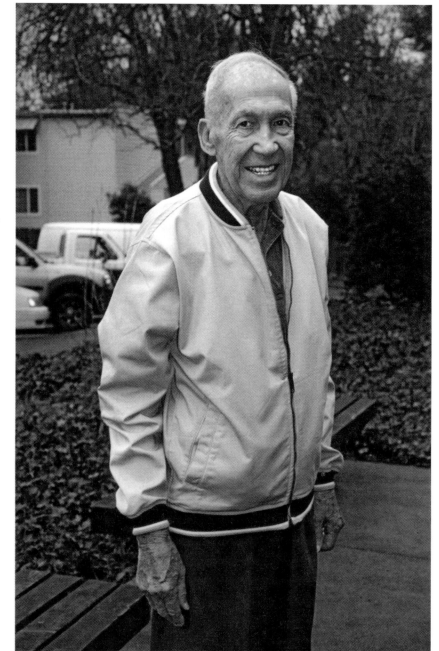

Howard

EIGHTY-TWO

I was born in Mt. Vernon, South Dakota. I grew up with
five brothers and four sisters, sharing a small five-room
house with no running water and an outhouse.

I attended grammar school and high school in Mitchell,
South Dakota. I was a very active, athletic child,
playing on three different sport teams. Fresh out of high
school I got a job with United Airlines, working there
forty-two years.

The love of my life, Violet, and I got married on October
26, 1946. We were married for fifty years. I was widowed
in 1996.

I attended a Senior Health Fair recently. There was a table
set up for osteoporosis testing. It was here that I found out
that I had very low bone density, which meant I had osteoporosis. Like so many people, I had no idea I had osteoporosis. It came as a surprise to me because I had always
been an active person and even now, in my later years,
I still like to sail and kayak.

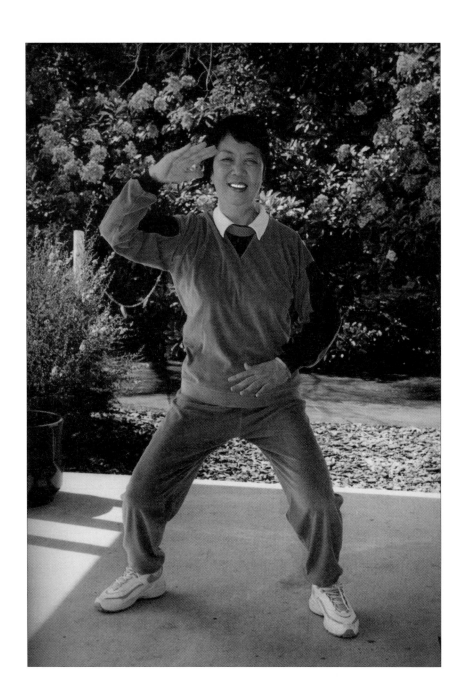

I am a retired registered nurse. I was born and grew up in China. Through my work I have seen patients with severe osteoporosis, some of whom got fractures while they were sleeping.

Being Chinese, I know that the Chinese don't like to drink milk. So our calcium intake is very poor. Most Asian women like to avoid sunlight in order to keep our skin soft and white. These attitudes contribute to our vitamin D level being low. I myself am tall with thin bones. Therefore, I know osteoporosis will get me sooner or later.

In September 1984, I fell and broke my leg and as a result had my first bone-density test. I was surprised to find out that osteoporosis had started on me so early. I was only 50 years old. I started taking calcium and exercising. Ten years later I had another bone-density test. I couldn't believe what I saw. The result was worse than ten years ago, even though I had been taking calcium supplements and exercising. My doctor prescribed hormone replacement therapy six years later, and my bone density then showed some improvement. Since hormone therapy may cause some side effects later on in life, my doctor suggested a change. In 2003, I started to use drug therapy and calcium together, and I have continued this therapy to the present.

I am now retired, which gives me a lot of time to exercise. I play table tennis three times a week. I also do Lu Tung Kuen, a Chinese exercise, daily, and teach Lu Tung Kuen twice a week. As if that weren't enough, I walk and go to the whirlpool.

After I joined the volunteer group, Foundation for Osteoporosis Research and Education (FORE), I learned to take calcium fifteen minutes after meals and only 500–600 mg each time. I also learned that our bodies cannot absorb excessive doses of calcium. I am very glad that FORE can constantly teach me new knowledge about osteoporosis and I can share this information with others. I hope by learning more about this disease, I can prevent its further progression both for me and for others.

Edith instructs Naifug in LuTung Kuen at the Chinese Senior Center. Naifug who is eighty-five also believes in taking control of her osteoporosis.

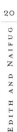

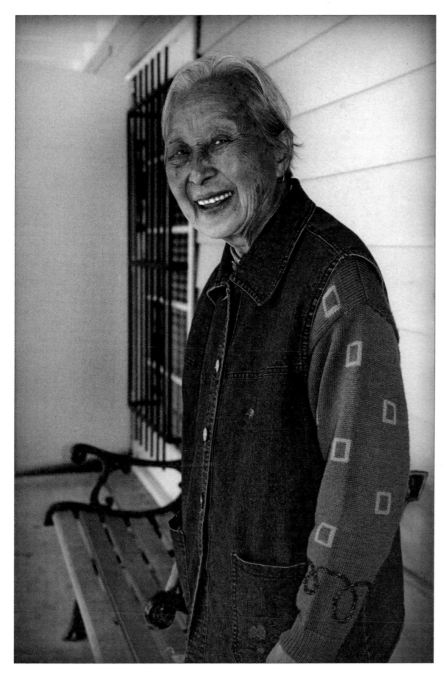

Neifug is happy to have Edith as an advocate
who is a voice for those in the Asian community.

Tonya

In January 2001, I was taking a group of seniors from Merrill Gardens to the Longs Drug Store in San Ramon to get their free bone-density test. My ladies from the retirement community had their tests, and then the technician asked if I would like to have my wrist tested.

I thought, of course, thinking that I would pass with flying colors. I had early menopause (46), but I am very active and have had cottage cheese or yogurt for lunch almost every day for years. However, I am Caucasian, small-framed and have never weighed more than 120 lbs. until the last five years. Now I am 58 and weigh 125 lbs. and am five foot four. I have been taking hormone replacement therapy for the last ten years. They explained to me my results. I scored very low and already had osteopenia and osteoporosis. I was shocked!

Anyway, I got the test results and they forwarded them to my doctor. I was 53 when I had my first wrist X-ray. My T-score is 1.9 standard deviations below the peak mean of young normal controls, indicating osteopenia. My physician immediately started me on drug therapy (one pill per week) and I increased my calcium. I started drinking orange juice with calcium, and started adding milk to my coffee (50% milk). I also included a slice of cheese in my sandwich on a daily basis. After two years, I was retested and my overall bone density increased 6%. I am very pleased with the results and so thankful that I took the time to be tested.

Looking back, I wish I had known how easy it was to get tested and I wish I had been tested at the onset of menopause to get a baseline reading. Also, I regret not drinking milk in my teenage years. I drank Diet Coke—tons of it! It is so easy to include calcium in your diet, especially since it is now available in so many different forms.

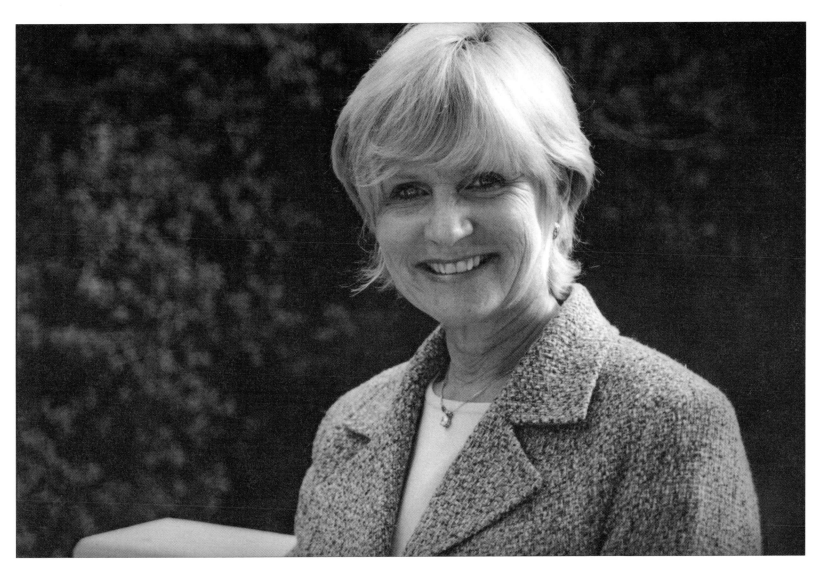

Tonya wanted to be in this book to help raise awareness about screening for osteoporosis.

Ruthie

My hope for you when you read this story is that you will learn that agony can turn into victory.

Like many people visiting Hawaii I didn't have a clue about the dangers of body surfing, but one day in my forties I was hit by two large waves, which tossed me in the air with amazing force. Landing on the sand with crashing force, my back was injured, and this changed my life.

The pain was constant and intolerable, and my search for help around the Bay Area where I live was extended all over the country. I had surgeries, went to pain centers for three weeks at a time, and had numerous treatments of all kinds.

My orthopedic surgeon insisted that morphine was the only drug that could help relieve the pain. For seventeen years, mega-doses of injectable morphine were prescribed, plus oral morphine. Much of that time I was bedridden, able to lie only on my back, with a caregiver and a bedpan. Needless to say, I ended up with osteoporosis as the lack of exercise for all those years contributed to a major loss of bone density, and at one point my weight was reduced to 89 lbs. I could find no answer to my plight, and felt desperate, confused, and alone.

I had severe episodes of anaphylactic shock, plus excruciating urinary tract pain from all the medication, and I had become a wretched shell of a woman.

My son, Adam, who was eight when I was injured, has since became a chiropractor. In desperation, I turned to Adam for help. Adam required me to have chiropractic treatments, exercise daily, eat organic and raw food, have periodic detoxification, and develop a positive mental attitude to help me recover. To my amazement, over time this healthy way of living my life worked!

My daily routine is to walk briskly for one to one and a half hours, using hills and stairs as much as possible, and to do at least a half-hour of strengthening and stretching exercises with weights and cables. Now, I am learning salsa, and have never felt so vital, joyful, and energetic.

It has been nearly nine years since I changed my way of living and thinking. With exercise and a positive attitude I expect my bones to last as long as I do!

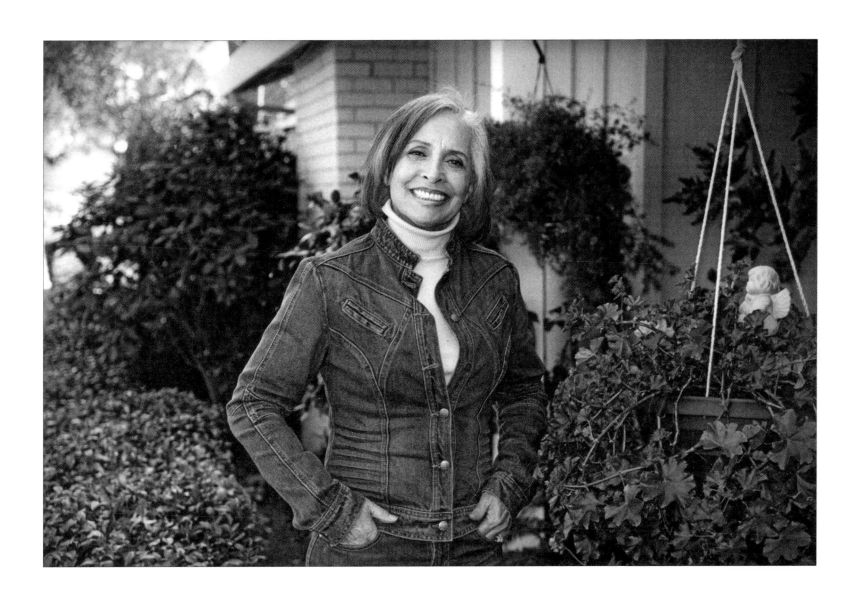

Joe, like Howard, was diagnosed with osteoporosis on this very day.

Joe

SEVENTY-EIGHT

I am 78 years young. My wife, Margaret, and I are con-
tinuing our honeymoon of thirty-two years. Together
we have five children (three daughters and two sons from
previous marriages), and ten grandchildren. I describe
myself in five ways. I'm a believer, family man, volunteer,
have a great sense of humor, and am easy to get along with.
I am active in the Napa Valley Senior Center, volunteer-
ing to serve in the lunch program. I participated in the
health screening for osteoporosis at the Napa Center and
will share the results with my doctor. After more than forty
years with Sears Roebuck and Company, I am enjoying
my retirement to the fullest extent.

Having overcome so many obstacles in her life, Yolanda inspired me. She accepts her disease as a part of her life.

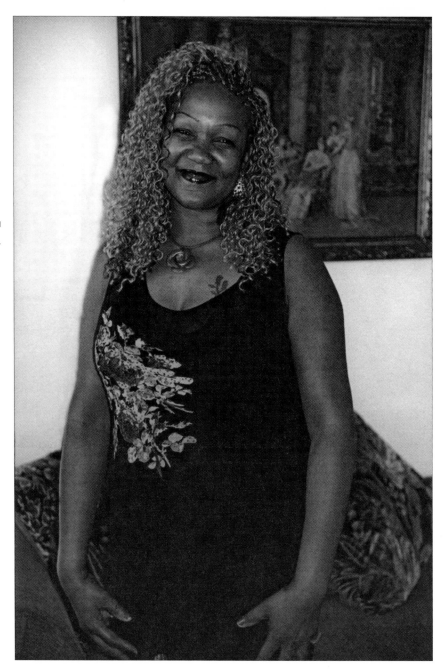

Yolanda

I remember when I was a little girl that I loved milk. My mother used to say I must think that my daddy was a cow. My daddy made sure that we kept milk in the house all the time. I am the youngest girl of my siblings—three girls and two boys.

As far back as I can remember I've battled pain, joint pain. I was diagnosed with sickle cell trait and hypertension, and arthritis as a child. I was not allowed to take physical education class, and there were limits to the physical activities I could do. I remember taking medicine all the time, and by the time I was thirteen I was a mother. At the age of nineteen I was a mother with two children and at the age of twenty-four I was the mother of three children. Now I have ten grandchildren. I take care of two of them full-time and most of them I see regularly. I am certified to take care of special-needs children and at the end of the day those children take care of me. They massage my legs and feet.

This year I was diagnosed with osteoporosis and high blood pressure. I take lots of medication for both. Over the years I've had some other battles, with drugs and men. My family and friends have always been my support, along with singing gospel and dressing up, to motivate me to press on past the constant pain. I thank God for the many opportunities as I continue to move forward. I have good days and bad days. On the bad days I don't want to get out of bed because of the pain. But I am a survivor and I don't let the bad days stop me from living my life.

I think about all the blessings God has given me and all the gifts of life. I'm in the studios recording my gospel music, and my dream is to someday adopt some more children to help care for. I just want to sing, look good, and share with the world the beauty that life can bring, and that the greatest gift is love, which I continue to share with others.

Kristi

I'm 34 years old, the youngest of seven children. I'm a Caucasian female, with blonde hair, blue eyes, and small-framed at five feet three. I have a family history of osteoporosis . . . and all of the risk factors for being a candidate.

I was diagnosed with osteopenia three years ago. I must say, I was not shocked.

I was athletically involved in different types of sports during my whole adolescence, and my parents made sure we always ate very healthy meals. As far back as I can recall, I don't remember ever hearing or being taught about the importance of taking care of my bones . . . but wow, was it important to brush your teeth!

My mother was diagnosed with osteoporosis eight years ago at the age of 64. She fell and crushed her kneecap while walking across a parking lot. Unfortunately, at that time, my mom did not get the best treatment or education about this debilitating bone disease. She was not put on osteo medications, but only told by her physician that she just needed to get more calcium in her diet. She also was not screened for osteoporosis.

Five years later, my parents were celebrating their fiftieth wedding anniversary with all seven of us kids, grandchildren, and great grandchildren. My mom went home that night and while getting ready for bed, she turned to reach up for her nightgown, heard a loud crack, and then fell to the floor. Unfortunately, the whole group was together again, only it was the hospital this time. Mom broke her hip and cracked her femur bone in two places. She did recover quite well with much hard work and devotion, which I couldn't imagine her not doing after bearing seven children.

To this day I choose to follow a healthy lifestyle. I eat healthy food, take multivitamins and calcium, exercise at least three times a week, don't smoke, and drink socially on occasion. But most important, I educate myself about this disease. I will never leave it up to someone else to give me enough information so that I can lead the healthiest life possible. I will always care about my teeth, but it is the bone that gives my teeth a place to shine.

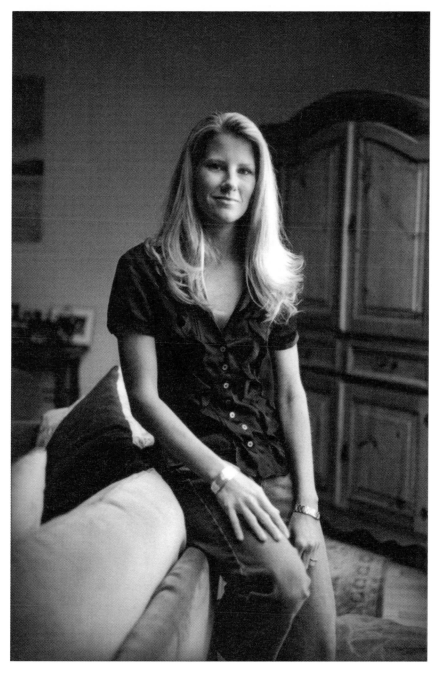

I know you are just as surprised as I am. Kristi is 35 with osteoporosis.

Carlos E. Torrese, M.A., M.DIV.

SPEAKS FOR THE LATINO COMMUNITY

"I was thinking that doctors will take some piece of my bone and that it will be a painful and traumatic test-screening, but it was very simple, not painful, so I know that I need to take care of myself, pay attention to my daily diet and tell my daughters and granddaughters that they need to have bone-density screenings." –Juan

Three years ago when the Senior Support Group received a visit from the Foundation for Osteoporosis Research and Education (FORE) to educate seniors and their caregivers about osteoporosis, the audience expressed their satisfaction at having this opportunity. For almost all of them this was the first time to have a bone-density test. It is "never too late to check my bones for the first time," said Maria, a 78-year-old woman who delivered twenty sons and daughters. She married sixty-three years ago and certainly she was very young. To the surprise of the group she was not at risk after the test. Juana, a 66-year-old woman with eight children, expressed her surprise, "Why am I at high risk? I don't have many children like Maria . . . . Now I know that I need to take care of my bones."

In communities where Latino seniors have limited access to health education, information, and orientation to using the health care system, support groups create a space for seniors to learn. A support group provides the opportunity for agencies like FORE and other professional providers to help underserved people get access to education and health screenings. Many seniors like Juan and Jose and their caregivers share this new experience, saying, "I was thinking that doctors will take some piece of my bone and that it will be a painful and traumatic test-screening, but it was very simple, not painful, so I know that I need to take care of myself, pay attention to my daily diet and tell my daughters and granddaughters that they need to have bone-density screenings." "Delivering the message around the community is the key. They changed their view and learned that they can practice prevention of this silent disease called osteoporosis," says Mr. Carlos Torres, coordinator of the Latino education and outreach programs of Jewish Family and Children's Services (JFCS) of the East Bay.

As part of the health education program, seniors and their caregivers learn that one out of two women and one out of eight men over fifty will suffer a fracture because of osteoporosis. Other facts indicate that osteoporosis affects more women than breast cancer, uterine cancer, and colon cancer combined. Osteoporosis can lead to debilitating hip fractures, vertebral fractures, and wrist fractures, according to FORE. The good news is that it is possible to prevent and treat bone loss and osteoporosis. If we take action today, we can improve bone health for a lifetime. With the help of the Osteoporosis Foundation, collaborating with Jewish Family and Children's Service's culturally and linguistically appropriate local programs, we are reaching out to underserved and disadvantaged Latino communities. Carlos Torres, JFCS staff and a member of the FORE speaker's bureau, hopes that "other health providers will be aware that education, information and follow-up, especially with limited English speakers who may be unfamiliar with osteoporosis, are necessary to prevent accidents and promote awareness about bone health in aging people, and to help achieve a better quality of life for underserved seniors."

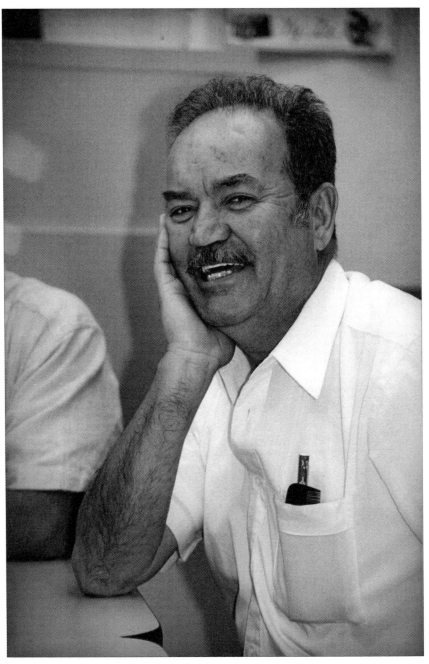

Santiago
SIXTY-NINE

Santiago shares a joke at the Senior Support Group.

Despite the language barrier and her economic hardship, Maria
wants to be educated about osteoporosis to share with her son.

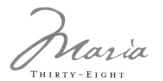

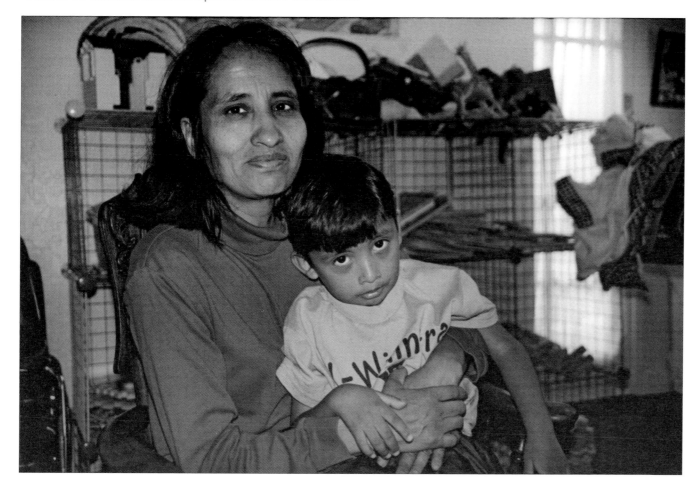

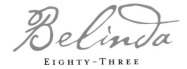

THIRTY-EIGHT

Belinda

EIGHTY-THREE

Belinda at the Bay Point Senior Support Group.

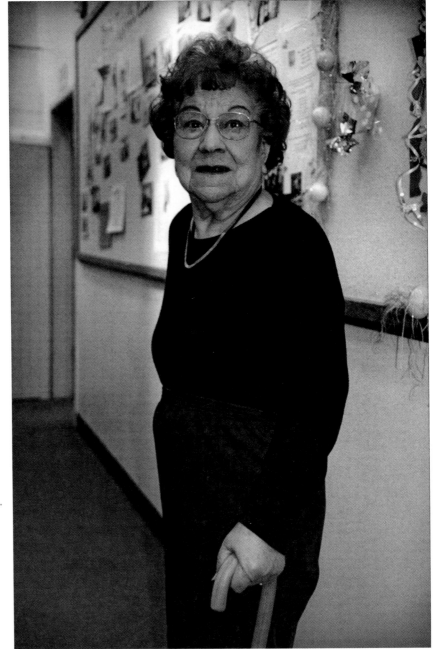

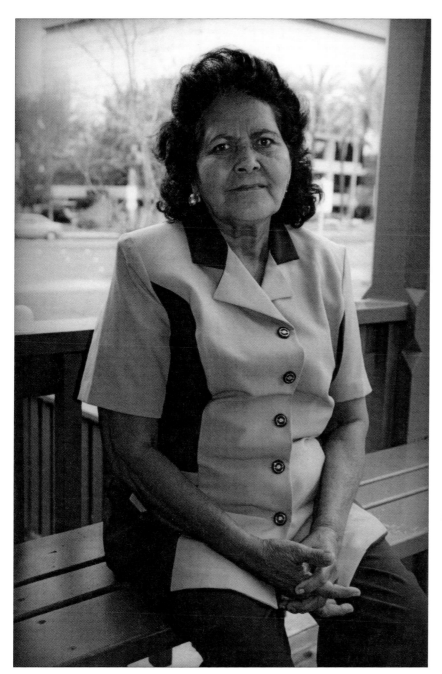

Rosario
SIXTY-EIGHT

Rosario outside the Latino Clinic.

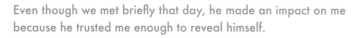

Giuadalupe

SIXTY-NINE

Even though we met briefly that day, he made an impact on me because he trusted me enough to reveal himself.

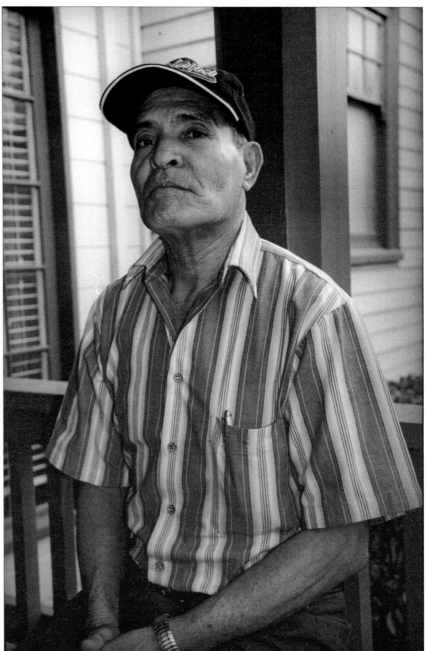

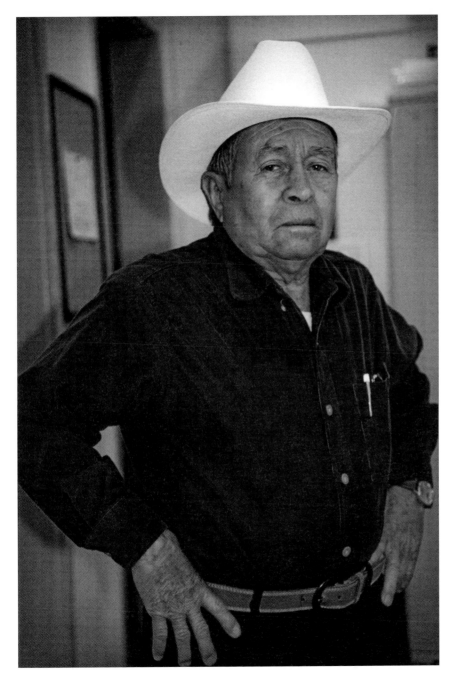

Juan
EIGHTY

Despite his proud stance, Juan is active
in taking control of osteoporosis.

Randi
FIFTY

I can still remember my first fracture. It was June 1995. I was 39 years old, and a birthday well-wisher whisked me around and gave me a very gregarious bear hug. I never told him that two of my ribs were broken that night.

I asked my rheumatologist, who treated me for lupus, to order me a bone-density scan ASAP. I knew I was at risk for osteoporosis. My mother had the disease, I'm very petite, and I'm being tested with glucocorticoid therapy. My doctor was shocked at my degree of bone loss. It was up to me to make lifestyle changes. I started medication, exercised, took my calcium and wore *sensible shoes*. It's important to protect yourself from falls. As the years have passed my fractures have been fewer and fewer. I'm fighting osteoporosis one day at a time.

I was so shocked to find out that Randi is living with osteoporosis and lupus, while being so positive.

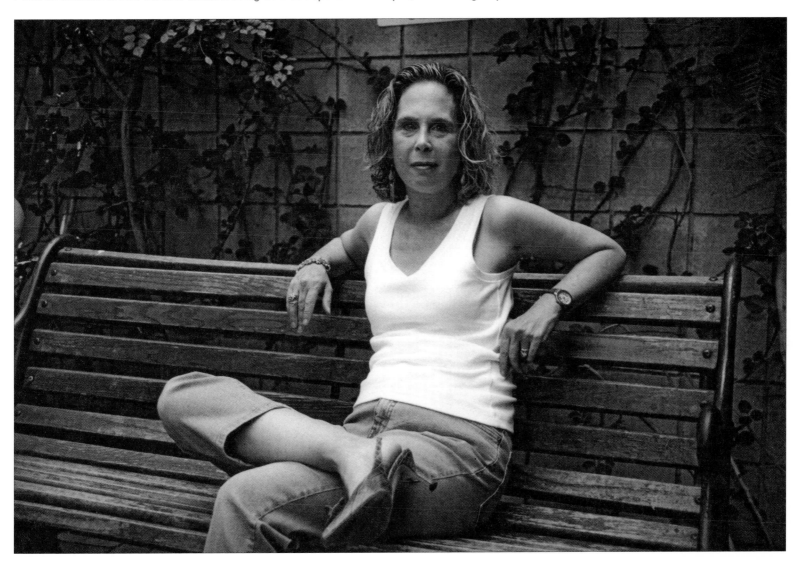

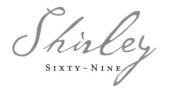

Shirley
SIXTY-NINE

I was born in a small town in North Carolina. I moved to Chicago, Illinois, at the age of 20. I was married and had two children.

One day in 1995, I stubbed my toe and went to the emergency room. The X-ray showed that not only did I have a fracture but I also had osteopenia. I was surprised because I have no family history of osteoporosis. The only medication the doctor gave me was calcium, 500 mg. two times a day. From then on, I was always careful, trying not to get another fracture. I never got another one.

Then in 2002 I moved to California. After going to a doctor there, I was sent to get a bone-density test. The test showed I have osteopenia. My doctor then started me on Fosamax. I take one pill very week. My doctor also increased my calcium to 1500 mg. a day.

A month ago I had another bone-density test, which showed that I still have osteopenia but it did not progress.

Sometimes I have aches and pains, but a Tylenol relieves the pain. I am on an exercise program; I walk seven days a week, about one and a half miles a day. I also have an exercise class I attend on Thursdays. I eat vegetables, fruit, fish, and chicken.

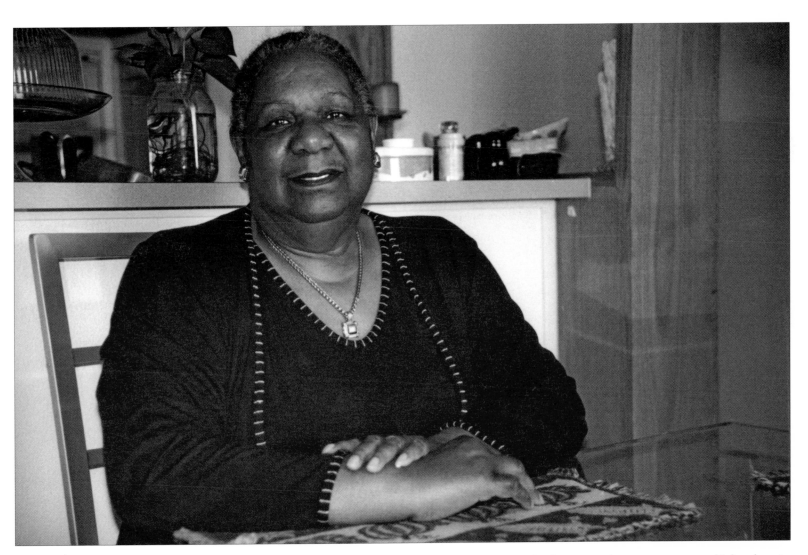

Shirley invited me into her home to share her story and I was interested to find out that her son and I share something in common, multiple sclerosis.

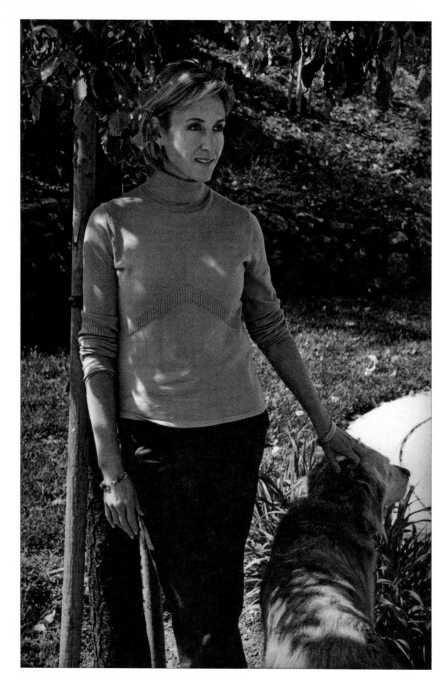

Perry Ann is such a vibrant and alive woman.

Osteoporosis—a disease for older people. Or so I thought.
I've done thousands of weight-bearing reps in the gym;
I've climbed many mountains, including a few of the high-
est peaks in North America and northern Europe; I've rid-
den 2,500 miles on my bike in Europe; I play tennis; I do
Pilates; I'm young; I eat a healthy diet; I've never smoked;
I take vitamins; and I've never broken a bone. So my bones
are healthy, right?

When my friend, past chairman of the Foundation for
Osteoporosis Research and Education (FORE), suggested
I, at then age 35, have a free bone-density test (hip and
spine) to help train technicians, I said, "Sure!" thinking
I was helping them more than they would be helping me.
Much to my surprise, my bones weren't as strong as I had
thought.

In fact, my results show that I fall into the osteopenia
range, indicating low bone mass and a possible precursor
to osteoporosis. Yes, I'm a woman; yes, I'm small-boned;
and yes, I'm fair-haired and fair-skinned, all risk factors

for osteoporosis, but I assumed my lifestyle choices over the years would have countered those predispositions. So what gives?

Two possible answers. First, genetics. At 66, my mother's tests are not indicative of osteoporosis; however, I'm convinced, even in the absence of tests, that my grandmother had the disease, given her hunched-over posture in her later years. Genetics, unfortunately, are out of my control.

Second, childhood diet. As a child, I didn't like milk much. I poured it over cereal, but was not a fan of drinking it by the glass. Since my osteopenia diagnosis, I've learned that 95% of one's bone mass is built before the age of 18, the very years I was not taking in as much calcium as I am now. The remaining 5% of bone mass is made between the ages of 18–28, the years I had taken a keen interest in my health, but I had missed that great opportunity during the earlier years to set the stage for strong health for the rest of my life.

Now I have two kids, four and six, and am highly alert to the fact that the calcium they take in through the food I feed them will benefit them for the rest of their lives.

What am I doing from here on to preserve my bone density? I'm now working with a bone specialist to establish a comprehensive baseline of my bone health. My blood tests show that my absorption of calcium is sufficient. So I will continue taking calcium through food and supplements. My vitamin D absorption is currently being tested. The specialist prescribed 55,000 IUs of the vitamin per week during the low-sun winter months. We'll do another bone-density test and vitamin absorption test in a few months to see how I'm doing. We'll go from there. Of course, I'll continue all of those beneficial lifestyle choices.

Now, at only 40, I'm very aware of maintaining my bone health and doing what I can to minimize and slow future loss. I fully intend to take after my parents and be active my entire life, especially when I'm older and have grandkids of my own. And I need strong bones to do it!

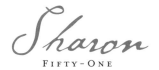

Sharon

FIFTY-ONE

The first time I realized I had a bone-density problem was at the young age of 34. I was on my annual family ski trip to Mammoth Lakes when I fell while I was skiing a fairly simple slope. The level of pain that followed was extraordinary, and I later was told that I had fractured two vertebrae in my back due to the fall. I realized that kind of result from a relatively nonserious accident was abnormal, but I neglected to seek treatment or investigate further what the problem was. It wouldn't be until sixteen years later, after I was elected an assemblywoman, that I would know why I had a history of easily fracturing my bones.

I was elected to represent the 36th Assembly District in November 2002. When I assumed office in January 2003, I realized an important part of my role as an assemblywoman was to learn about a variety of new issues I had little experience with before that time. Many groups help new legislators learn about their issues by having various events here at the state capitol. One such event is a bone-density screening provided to legislators and staff to learn more about osteoporosis. Knowing that I might have a problem, I went out to get the test and learn more about osteoporosis. After my bone-density test yielded abnormal results for my age, doctors at the screening suggested that I see my doctor to get a full screening.

I went to see my doctor, and he confirmed that I have very low bone density for my age and suffer from osteoporosis.

He immediately put me on medication to help me with my osteoporosis. However, I stopped the treatment almost immediately because the medication made me feel very ill all day after I ingested the pill. Since there are limited options to treat osteoporosis I no longer take a prescription drug to treat the condition but rather take calcium supplements and vitamins.

I remember as a child and through my teens and twenties I never drank milk and did not eat any high-calcium foods. I realize now that had I properly addressed my family history with osteoporosis earlier in my life I might have been able to save myself from many of the symptoms I now experience. Now I make sure that my 17-year-old daughter and 28-year-old son know about our family history and address the issue accordingly.

My doctor has informed me that a new medication that treats osteoporosis will be coming out in the near future. I look forward to trying that treatment and hope it does not produce the negative side affects I experienced with other medications. Regardless of family history or lack of symptoms, I think it is important for people, especially women, to get the simple bone-density test no matter what age you are. The earlier you know there is a problem, the earlier you can treat it, and the better off you will be in the long run.

46

SHARON

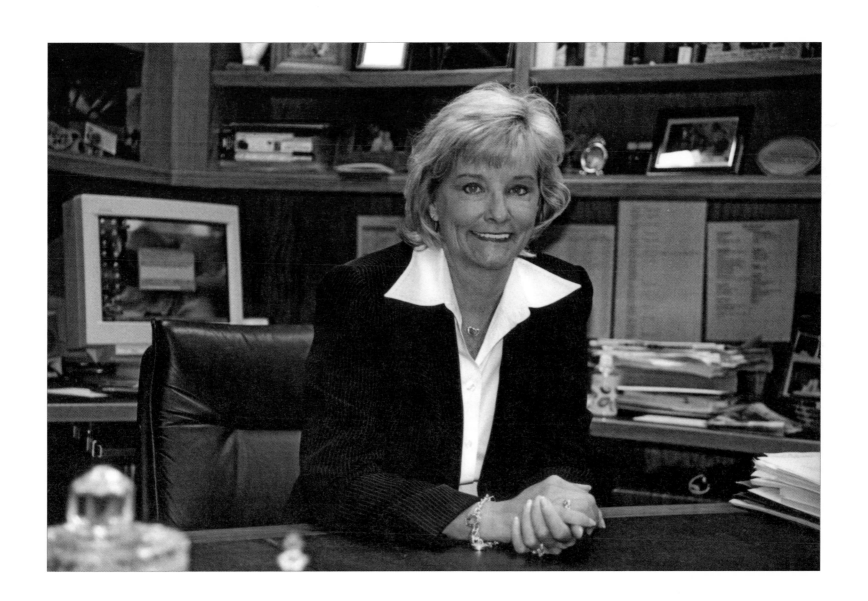

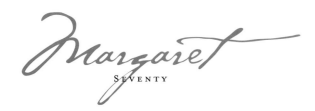

Margaret

SEVENTY

I was born in Los Angeles on April 10, 1935. We were raised in the Bay Area. I graduated from high school in 1954, but married in 1953. Had two miscarriages in 1954 and 1955, separated from my husband in 1955. I moved to the L.A. area and went to college at UCLA for two years. I came back to the Bay Area and joined the Marine Corps in 1957–1962.

I had always had very bad monthly periods. In late 1962 I was in the hospital for endometriosis and had my left tube and appendix removed. I was working for Hughes Aircraft in Engineering. The pain and periods still were very bad in 1967, so I went back to the doctor, and this time I had cancer. They removed the other tube, the uterus, ovary, and some intestines. They said I would be on medication for the rest of my life. I told them I could live with hot flashes. Little did I know that when I turned 50 my bones would start to ache and I finally had to give up tennis. The hysterectomy started me into menopause and osteoporosis. But I lived with it. In 1986 my right hip had a plate put in, and the bone rejected the metal so they put in a replacement. The hip rejected that, but they couldn't do anything with that so they said live with it. I had also very bad backaches and my bones ached all the time. They said I had curvature of the spine and osteoarthritis. They gave me medicine but nothing helped.

So, since 1986 I have been in pain. My bones are brittle, and now on my seventieth birthday there still is nothing I can do but as they have always said, live with the pain. The bones rejected the medications. So I pray a lot and keep busy as much as possible.

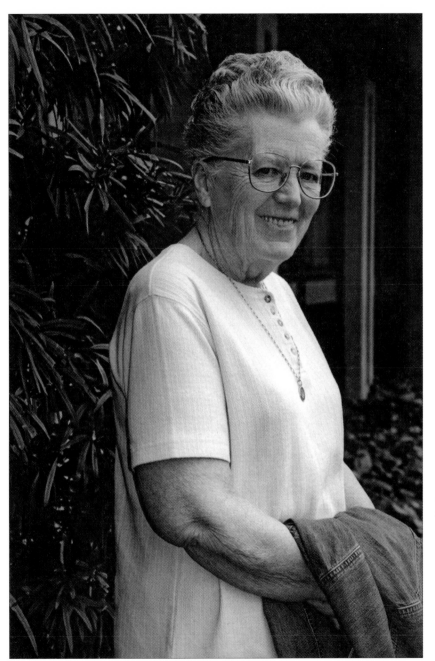

Margaret is very positive for finding
out she has osteoporosis.

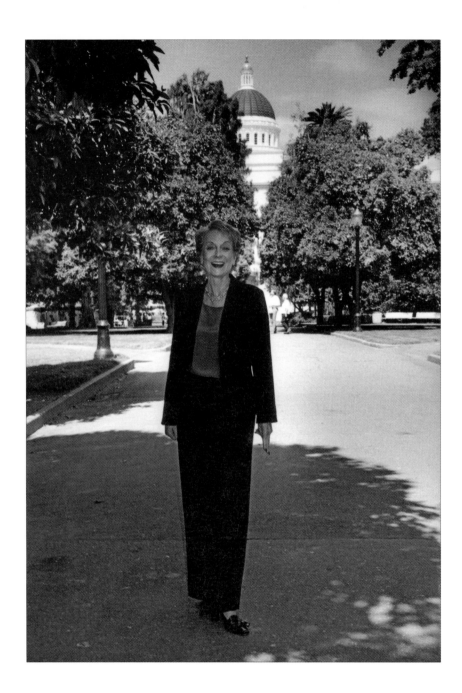

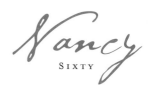

In 1983, I was a happy, healthy, 38-year-old single mom raising a fabulous six-year-old daughter. I had a job I loved, a family who loved me unconditionally, and lots of wonderful friends.

Then in May, I found a lump in my breast. By the end of the month, I had been told I had breast cancer and because of its advanced stage, I might have two years to live. I made a decision that day to not allow the disease to be more than a minor inconvenience in my life, and I told the doctors that they only "practiced" medicine, and that I would defer to a Higher Power with regard to my destiny. I had surgery, radiation therapy, and chemotherapy. I worked, meditated, loved my daughter, kept only positive thoughts, laughed with my friends and lived my life.

Twelve years later, during my yearly oncology "wellness" check, I mentioned that I might be at risk for osteoporosis (not realizing at the time that the radiation and chemotherapy I had undergone were factors as well). My oncologist agreed and referred me to an endocrinologist who said she wasn't sure I was at risk since I had no family history, but ordered a bone-density test because it would give us a baseline reading for future use.

The day after the test, I received a call from the doctor asking if I would come in that afternoon to discuss the results. The test showed I had more than a 33% loss of bone. At the age of 50 my bones were determined to be those of an 89-year-old woman. I was started on various methods of therapy to try and rebuild bone, including trial medications and daily injections of calcitonin.

In the meantime, I began my own research. At age 38, my first chemotherapy treatment had sent me directly into menopause. For years I experienced unbelievable hot flashes and night sweats. But because my cancer was hormone-induced, I was told I would never be able to take hormone replacement therapy (HRT) to counter the effects. I consulted with doctors who studied this subject, one in particular at the M.D. Anderson Cancer Institute in Houston, Texas, and made my own personal decision to ask for HRT. After months of discussions with my oncologist, endocrinologist, and obstetrician, it was agreed that I could begin minimal HRT. Soon afterwards, a new bone-building product came out on the market called Fosamax and it was prescribed for me. After being on this new drug and HRT for two years, I underwent another bone-density test. The results indicated I had gained significant bone. I am still taking HRT and drug therapy, and my last bone-density test showed that my bones were those of a 65-year-old woman. I am thrilled and I am truly blessed.

Years ago, I chose quality of life over quantity of life. I am 60 this year, newly married, still thinking positively and still living life to the fullest. These are my choices—and ones I plan to continue for many, many years to come!

Sarah

"Wait," I demanded of my boyfriend, "they're doing free bone-density tests; it'll just take a few minutes." We were at a health fair, checking out the booths and collecting free samples. When it was my turn, I placed my heel in the machine and waited anxiously for my little printout. At 21 years old I was quite the narcissist. "I'm three times younger than anyone else in line, I go to the gym five days a week, and I run half-marathons. My score is going to be the best!" I thought to myself.

When the physician finished explaining that my T-score was actually quite low, I waited for her to tell me that the machine seemed to be generating false readings. Instead she suggested that I see my doctor for a more thorough exam. "These volunteers don't know what they're doing!" I insisted, too quietly to be heard. Or maybe this was another scam—like those chiropractors who falsely diagnose everyone with scoliosis so they can get more patients. But when no one tried to sell me magic pills or special therapy, I came to the unfortunate realization that this might be serious.

My doctor reluctantly prescribed the DEXA scan I requested, but not without humiliating me by undermining my intelligence and suggesting I was a hypochondriac. Unfortunately, my concerns were justified when the specialist called with my results—"I've never seen such a severe case in someone so young before." As I hung up the phone I felt like I had just been robbed of my sanctuary. It took some time to mend my psyche, but soon I became committed to a lifestyle of recovery. This meant doing everything possible to increase bone mass. My doctor told me to engage in as many weight-bearing activities as possible, which was easy enough since I had been lifting weights for years. I was also told to consume plenty of calcium and take supplements every day, which was also manageable—who doesn't like cheese and ice cream? Lastly, my doctor prescribed a bisphosphonate, medication I take, but with much apprehension. When he asked if I had heard of the medication, I told him "Yeah, I've seen the commercials. They advertise it during Wheel of Fortune, in between the ads for Viagra and Depends." Besides the indigestion that the pills cause, there is another concern of mine—there have been no studies on this drug's effect on young populations. Even today all clinical trials mandate that participants be post-menopausal or older than 50. I guess this means that I'm the guinea pig.

I've now been aware of my "low bone density," this being the official term since pre-menopausal woman cannot be branded as having "osteoporosis," for over five years. I try to live each day as if tomorrow I could be hospitalized with a broken hip or fractured vertebrae. I follow an intense workout regimen, take my medications and try to remain

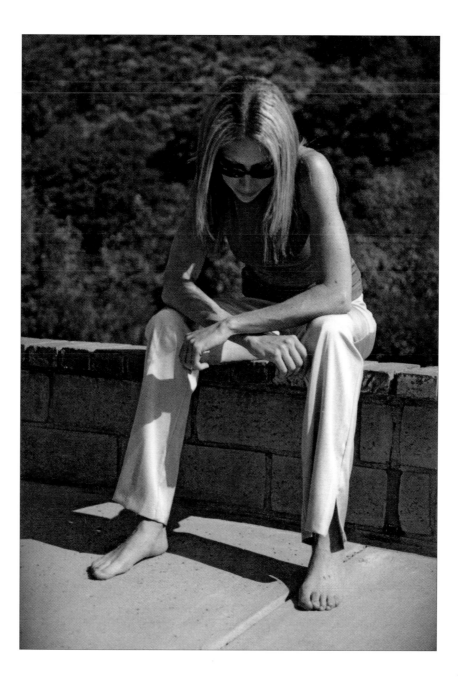

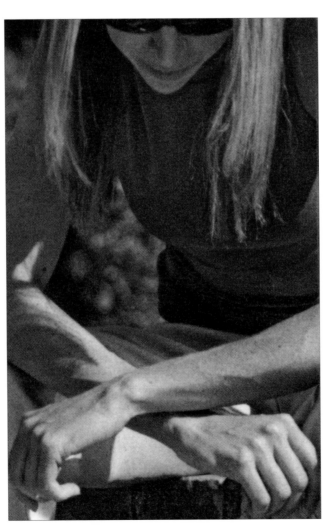

hopeful for a cure. Honestly, though, I do have those moments of self-pity. I can't enjoy a soda or an alcoholic beverage with friends without thinking about how it is robbing my body of calcium. And whenever I see an elderly person, hunchbacked, gaze now permanently fixed to the floor, I see myself in a just few years. It is then that I cry inside.

Partly because of pride, but more because of the ignorant and often disparaging environment in which we live, I rarely reveal my condition to others. While on a hike I once told a man I was dating about my bones. He wanted to carry me back to our car in case I fell, and then he asked, "If we have sex, will I break you?" Of course, this silence does nothing for spreading awareness or changing society's perspective; and so I share my story here.

Well, if you've read this far perhaps you have enough interest to tolerate a little preaching. My message is this: low bone density is not just an "old person's" disease. It is a problem that affects kids with rheumatoid arthritis and patients undergoing cancer therapy. Severely weakened bones are seen in anorexic and bulimic teens and in young athletes, too. It is never too early to eat healthy and build strong bones, and you and your children are never too young to be tested for a life-threatening disease. After all, you can't improve a condition without knowing how to treat it or without being aware that it exists in the first place.

Andrew

Andrew was nine years old when diagnosed with osteoporosis. We found out about his osteoporosis when a swing he was swinging on at school broke. He was taken by ambulance to the hospital. Andrew was in a lot of pain but so brave. I remember him lying there on a backboard and neck brace right in front of the nurse's station where we waited all day for someone to help him. I overheard a nurse say to another nurse that Andrew was O.K., just bruised. No big deal. When the X-ray technician finally came, he too was quite rough with Andrew, but I knew something was up because after taking the X-rays, the technician all of a sudden started to act concerned and was much gentler with Andrew. It turned out Andrew had three compression fractures in his back, and his bones showed that he had osteoporosis.

There has been no family member with any bone disease that we know of. Andrew's bone density test showed he was four standard deviations below where he should have been. It has been a great concern to his doctors. Andrew went through an operation for two skin biopsies and one bone biopsy to try to figure out why he has osteoporosis. The biopsies turned up no reason and his osteoporosis is still a mystery. He went through a two-year treatment at Children's Hospital with an infusion of Pomindoranate. We would spend a day at Children's Hospital with an IV four times a year. We keep our fingers crossed that this treatment will help stop the breaking down of his bones. Andrew cannot play any contact sports or anything that puts him at risk of falling. On top of the osteoporosis, Andrew also has Asperger's, which is high-functioning autism. All of this has changed Andrew's life, and the doctors don't know why any of this happened. In spite of this, Andrew handles it all very well, and I am so proud of him.

ANDREW

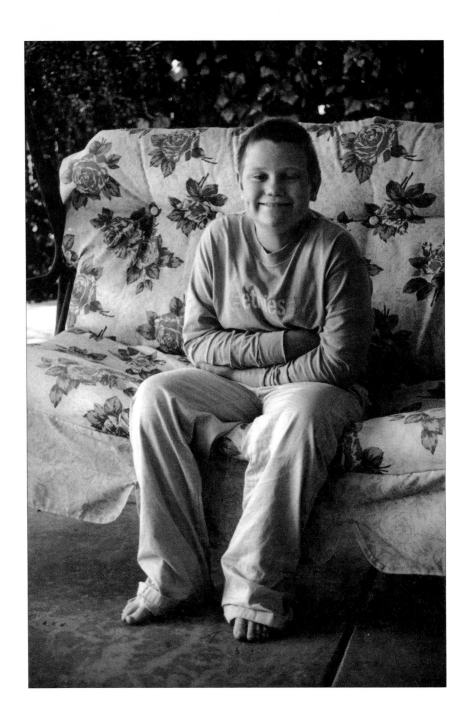

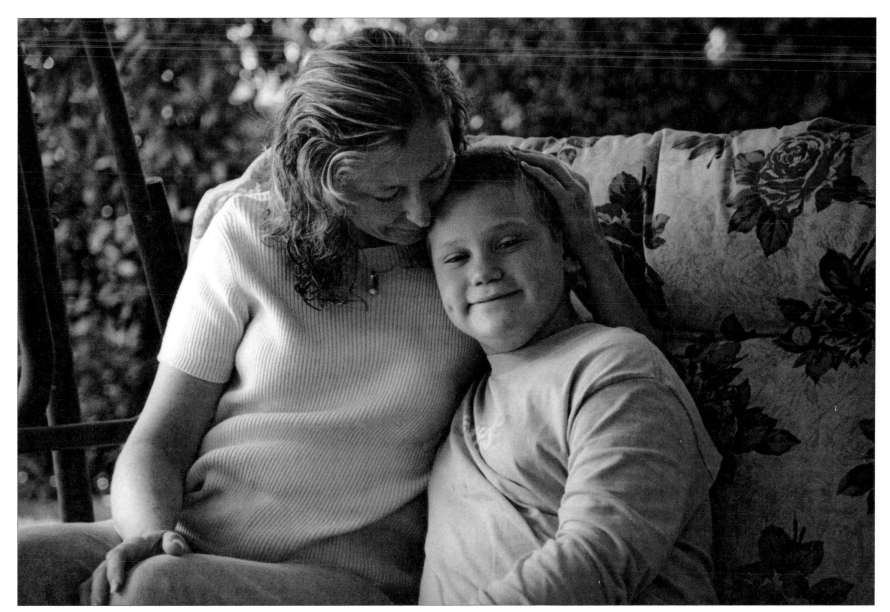

ANDREW

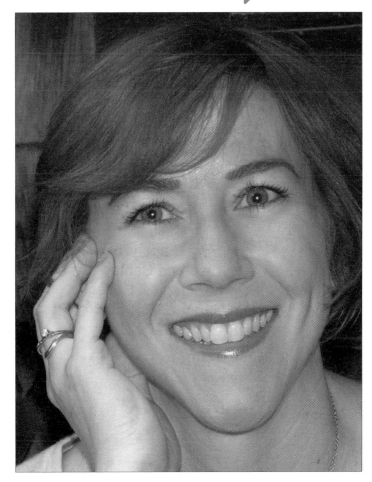

Amelia Davis is an award-winning photographer. She has shown her work in fine art galleries, at universities, and at medical symposiums including The Society for Contemporary Photography in Kansas City (MO), the Hang Gallery in San Francisco, and the California Breast Cancer Research Symposium. Amelia's photographs have been seen in the *San Francisco Chronicle* and *American Photo* magazine. Her photographs deal with life's realities head-on. Amelia does not hide the truth; instead she allows the viewer to confront it.

Amelia has been a grant recipient for her photo documentary book about breast cancer survivors, *The First Look*, as well as for her last book, *My Story*, which shows people and their caregivers living with multiple sclerosis. Amelia was diagnosed with MS in 1998. She is President of The VisionWorks Foundation, Inc., a non-profit organization dedicated to patient-guided outreach. The first project of this foundation is MSFriends Initiative, a 24/7 helpline.

The First Look received The Sixteenth Annual Susan Koppelman Award for editing, and was selected by the AAUP Book and Jacket Show as one of the best-designed books of 2000.

Amelia has been a guest speaker at various fundraising events for breast cancer and multiple sclerosis and has appeared on T.V. and radio shows, such as PBS's "Forum."